Domiziana Santucci
Carlo de Felice

MRI and histological prognostic factors in breast cancer

AF138593

Domiziana Santucci
Carlo de Felice

MRI and histological prognostic factors in breast cancer

A study of the correlation between grading and ADC provided by DWI

LAP LAMBERT Academic Publishing

Impressum / Imprint

Bibliografische Information der Deutschen Nationalbibliothek: Die Deutsche Nationalbibliothek verzeichnet diese Publikation in der Deutschen Nationalbibliografie; detaillierte bibliografische Daten sind im Internet über http://dnb.d-nb.de abrufbar.

Alle in diesem Buch genannten Marken und Produktnamen unterliegen warenzeichen-, marken- oder patentrechtlichem Schutz bzw. sind Warenzeichen oder eingetragene Warenzeichen der jeweiligen Inhaber. Die Wiedergabe von Marken, Produktnamen, Gebrauchsnamen, Handelsnamen, Warenbezeichnungen u.s.w. in diesem Werk berechtigt auch ohne besondere Kennzeichnung nicht zu der Annahme, dass solche Namen im Sinne der Warenzeichen- und Markenschutzgesetzgebung als frei zu betrachten wären und daher von jedermann benutzt werden dürften.

Bibliographic information published by the Deutsche Nationalbibliothek: The Deutsche Nationalbibliothek lists this publication in the Deutsche Nationalbibliografie; detailed bibliographic data are available in the Internet at http://dnb.d-nb.de.

Any brand names and product names mentioned in this book are subject to trademark, brand or patent protection and are trademarks or registered trademarks of their respective holders. The use of brand names, product names, common names, trade names, product descriptions etc. even without a particular marking in this work is in no way to be construed to mean that such names may be regarded as unrestricted in respect of trademark and brand protection legislation and could thus be used by anyone.

Coverbild / Cover image: www.ingimage.com

Verlag / Publisher:
LAP LAMBERT Academic Publishing
ist ein Imprint der / is a trademark of
OmniScriptum GmbH & Co. KG
Heinrich-Böcking-Str. 6-8, 66121 Saarbrücken, Deutschland / Germany
Email: info@lap-publishing.com

Herstellung: siehe letzte Seite /
Printed at: see last page
ISBN: 978-3-659-78290-9

Zugl. / Approved by: Rome, University of Rome "La Sapienza", Diss., 2014

To my family and Ale,
real strength and inspiration of my life

Index

Figures and Tables

Abstract

The aim of this retrospective study was to evaluate whether the apparent diffusion coefficient (ADC) generated by ADC maps provided by 3.0 Tesla (3T) magnetic resonance imaging (MRI) including diffusion-weighted imaging (DWI) varied according to the histological grading of invasive breast carcinoma.

A total of 92 patients with 96 invasive breast cancer lesions were enrolled. All patients had undergone 3T MRI for local staging. All lesions detected at MRI were subsequently confirmed by histological analysis after surgery or core biopsy. The MRI protocol included contrast-enhanced sequences and DWI sequences; ADC value was calculated for each lesion on the basis of the obtained ADC map.

Histological tumor grade was established according to the Nottingham Grading System (NGS), and the lesions were divided into the following groups: G1, G2, G3.

ADC values which did not follow a normal distribution were compared with the grading using two nonparametric statistical tests: the Mann-Whitney U test and the Kruskal-Wallis H test. Spearman's Rho test was performed to correlate grading with other prognostic factors, such as tumor size, estrogen and progesterone receptor status, HER2 expression and Ki-67 index to determine the significance of grading alone in predicting tumor aggressiveness and to demonstrate the capability of grading to summarize histological prognostic factors

Pearson's chi square test was therefore carried out to compare the values obtained in the two extreme grading classifications (G1 and G3). The tests showed that ADC values were significantly higher in G1 than in G3 ($p < 0.05$) whereas no significant difference was observed when G1 and G3 were compared to G2.

In conclusion, ADC values obtained with 3T DWI sequences correlate with low and high histological grading in invasive breast carcinoma lesions. ADC seems to be a useful tool for identifying highly aggressive breast tumors and determining biological behavior to obtain more accurate prognostic information and guide therapeutic choices.

Introduction

After skin cancer, breast carcinoma is the most common malignancy in women. A woman who lives to the age of 90 has a 1 in 8 risk of developing breast cancer in her lifetime[1]. It is ironic and tragic that cancer affecting an organ such as the breast which is so easily accessible for clinical and diagnostic examination, continues to claim so many human lives.

Today, breast cancer is considered a heterogeneous disease with a wide variety of phenomena and histological aspects. In the past, it was customary to consider breast cancer as a homogeneous group of diseases, but today we know that histological factors determine important phenotypic variations which affect the prognosis including likelihood of recurrence and metastatic disease. This obviously influences the therapeutic planning and management.

It is therefore essential to identify type, biological behavior and histochemical features of breast cancer lesions through invasive histological or cytological procedures and non-invasive procedures, such as diagnostic imaging.

Mammography and ultrasound (US) imaging are conventional techniques, which have for many years been used in screening and diagnosis of breast lesions. More recently, additional techniques have been introduced in the evaluation and characterization of the lesions, such as magnetic resonance imaging (MRI) which has been found to have the highest sensitivity among the available imaging techniques, ranging between 88% and 95% [2-4]. However, several authors have reported a moderate specificity of traditional MRI including contrast enhanced T2- and T1-weighted sequences, ranging from 30% to 80% [2,5,6]. Moreover, sequences requiring injection of contrast medium may in rare cases cause side effects. For these reasons, ongoing research projects are focused on the development of techniques that increase the specificity of breast MRI while reducing the side effects linked to administration of contrast medium.

In particular, diffusion-weighted imaging (DWI) is a valid contribution to traditional sequences in the characterization of breast lesions. DWI is a fast and non-invasive technique which reveals the biological character of the Brownian motion of protons in bulk water molecules *in vivo*. This motion along three orthogonal axes can be measured quantitatively by evaluating the apparent diffusion coefficient (ADC) which reflects the structural properties of the tissues, cellularity, fluid viscosity, membrane permeability and blood flow[7-11].

The reduced mobility of water molecules in densely cellular tissues correlates with an increased signal restriction in DWI and a reduced ADC value, which is lower in malignant tumors with high proliferative activity. Assessment of malignancy which is required to guide the clinician towards the most appropriate therapeutic choices, takes numerous prognostic factors into account. Among these factors, one of the most important is histological grading, which is obtained by evaluating the morphological structure and some anatomopathological features of the lesion. Several authors have highlighted the close and direct relationship between grading and prognosis. Elston and Ellis thus reported that patients with grade 1 lesions had a better prognosis than patients with grade 2 or grade 3 lesions[12].

Also the morphohistological features of the lesion are evaluated to establish a prognosis, such as size, estrogen (ER) and progesterone (PgR) receptor status, human epidermal growth factor receptor 2 (HER2) and cell proliferation expressed by Ki-67 index.

Grading seems to correlate with these prognostic factors and can therefore provide important information and reveal the biological nature of the tumor[7].

Several studies have examined the relationship between ADC values and prognostic factors, including grading[11,13,14]. The aim of this study is to compare grading with ADC values obtained from DWI sequences in breast cancer lesions and to prove the importance of ADC as a prognostic factor through correlation with other histological features.

6

1. Role of MRI in breast cancer

Today MRI is considered the most accurate imaging technique in the assessment of breast cancer lesions. The diagnostic role of dynamic sequences after administration of gadolinium-based contrast medium has been particularly studied[2]. The use of this method has steadily increased over the years despite the lack of clear evidence of its effectiveness in many fields; only 11 meta-analyses have been conducted from 1995 to 2010[3].

The following indications for breast MRI in breast cancer are included in the guidelines issued by the European Society of Breast Cancer Specialists (EUSOMA) during the workshop in Milan in October 2008.

- **Screening of high-risk women**. Several genetic mutations predispose women to an increased risk of developing breast cancer. Approximately 3% of all breast cancers are linked to high-penetrance mutations in cancer-susceptibility genes, such as BRCA1 and BRCA2, tumor suppressor TP53 (Li Fraumeni syndrome) or moderate/low-penetrance allelic mutations, such as CHEK2, ATM e BRIP1.

BRCA mutation carries a 50% and 60% increased risk of developing breast and ovarian cancer, respectively, and regular MRI screening is therefore recommended. MRI screening is recommended also in women with Cowden, Li Fraumeni and Bannayan-Riley-Ruvalcaba syndromes and in women who have undergone radiotherapy for lung cancer before 30 years of age. In contrast, evidence is too insufficient to recommend MRI screening in women with lobular intraepithelial neoplasia, atypical ductal hyperplasia, elevated breast density at mammography and a personal history of breast cancer, including ductal carcinoma in situ[3].

- **Breast implants**. MRI is definitely more accurate than physical examination and traditional imaging for evaluating the integrity of breast implants inserted for cosmetic purposes or to assist cosmesis after surgical treatment of breast cancer. MRI is also the most sensitive technique for differentiating between intra- and extracapsular implant rupture and for evaluating the possible extension of silicone leakage and formation of granuloma. MRI is recommended in patients with symptoms suggesting breast implant rupture, in patients with signs and symptoms of initial or recurrent breast disease (e.g. breast cancer) in cases where conventional diagnostic methods yield unclear or negative outcome and in asymptomatic women with breast implants inserted for reconstructive purposes after surgery and with high risk of recurrence.

- **Pre-surgical staging**. Staging plays an important role in estimating prognosis and particularly in the therapeutic planning. The choice between conservative treatment, i.e. local excision or quadrantectomy and radiotherapy, and radical treatment, i.e. mastectomy, is essentially based on tumor size with 3 cm tumor diameter cutoff of the largest lesion and the presence of foci.

There are excellent data from single and multi-center studies that confirm the high sensitivity of MRI in the evaluation of lesion size and the identification of multifocal and multicentric tumors compared to the traditional imaging methods, mammography and breast US.

Sardanelli et al.[16] thus demonstrated a pre-surgical MRI sensitivity of 81% in detecting ductal carcinomas. Mann et al[4] reported a sensitivity of 93% in detecting lobular carcinomas, and the percentage increased when evaluation of multiple foci was included. Another important feature of MRI is the ability to identify also intraductal components.

Several authors have recognized that MRI has limitations owing to the rather low specificity in identifying malignant lesions, when using only pre- and post-contrast T2- and T1-weighted sequences[16]. This has emphasized the need for additional diagnostic investigation, such as second-look US or MRI-guided biopsy in case of injuries visible only on MRI.

-**Response to neo-adjuvant chemotherapy**. The purpose of neoadjuvant chemotherapy (NACT) is to reduce the size of the tumor in order to ensure the best possible result of local surgery. NACT is indicated in patients diagnosed with cancer which is inoperable at first presentation due to pectoral muscle, skin or nipple invasion or distant metastases. NACT is also administered in case of operable lesions of large dimensions (stages IIa, IIb and IIIa) that may not be indicated for conservative treatment. MRI provides the multidisciplinary team with the information required to decide on the most appropriate treatment, thanks to the ability of this diagnostic method to identify the true extension of the tumor after NACT administration.

In patients who are considered inoperable, MRI is performed at first presentation, and patients with large, potentially operable lesions are submitted to MRI before NACT, provided that MRI does not postpone the therapy. Post-NACT MRI is preferably performed two weeks after the last cycle of chemotherapy and two weeks before surgery.

Pre- and post-NACT evaluation includes concurrent assessment of the two MRI scans carried out to detect increased signal at the site of the tumor after administration of contrast medium. Measurement of residual disease was estimated according to the Response Evaluation Criteria in Solid Tumors (RECIST) or the World Health Organization (WHO) criteria.

- **Postsurgical follow-up.** Traditional imaging tests and/or clinical examination may suggest recurrence, as it may be difficult to distinguish between new lesions and postsurgical residual tumor. In these cases, MRI is useful due to the high diagnostic accuracy and sensitivity of this method in the detection of recurrence in the scar, ranging from 93% to 100%, and specificity ranging from 88% to 100%.

- **Cancer of unknown primary (CUP) syndrome or occult primary cancer.** About 1% of breast cancers are diagnosed thanks to signs and symptoms related to metastatic disease (lymph node metastasis) with no evidence of the primary tumor. In approximately 5% of cases, metastases are located in the axillary lymph nodes, and this together with high estrogen and progesterone receptor levels suggests the breast as the site of the primary tumor. In such cases, mammography identifies the tumor in about 33% of patients. However, when both mammography and US fail to detect a tumor that fine-needle aspiration or lymph node removal has confirmed, MRI is performed due to the high sensitivity and the ability to detect primary lesions in more than 50% of cases.

2. Contrast-enhanced MRI sequences

Contrast-enhanced MRI sequences are carried out after intravenous administration of contrast medium, and the advantage of this method is the high sensitivity and positive predictive value. It is currently considered as the most appropriate method in the assessment of breast cancer, thanks to the ability to solve diagnostic problems which remain unsolved after conventional clinical-diagnostic methods, such as mammography and US.

The contrast medium is a paramagnetic, gadolinium chelating substance that is injected into a vein, typically the brachial vein, during the examination. This substance spreads into the vascular space and then into the organs like the iodinated contrast media used in computed tomography (CT). The Gadolinium molecules temporarily alter the molecular properties of nearby water molecules within the magnetic field of the structures they enter, thereby changing the signal intensity of the tissues in a manner dependent on the local concentration of molecules. However, unlike CT this relationship is not linear[5].

Image acquisition includes:

- Depiction of a pre-contrast T1-weighted ($T1_0$ map) image, which will serve as a map for calculating contrast medium concentration;
- Acquisition of T1-weighted images during and after administration of contrast medium; a reasonably high temporal resolution allows evaluation of contrast medium wash-in and wash-out.

The obtained images show the distribution of contrast medium in the tissues. This distribution is more evident and more easy to interpret in the "subtracted" sequences, i.e. images that are obtained by "subtracting" the $T1_0$ map, which acts as a mask, from the images acquired after the bolus of contrast medium has reached the region of interest (ROI).

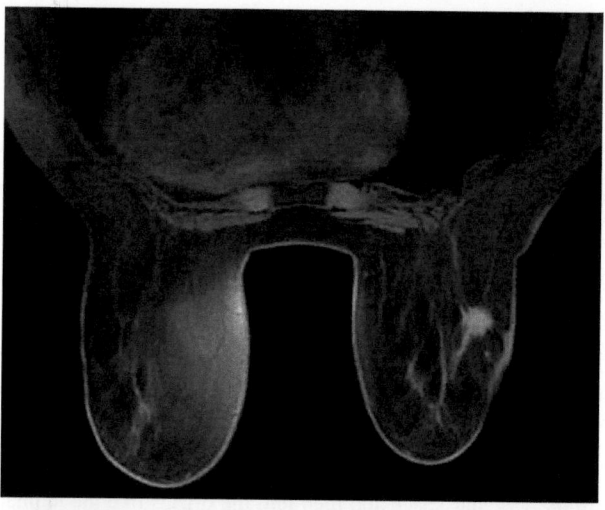

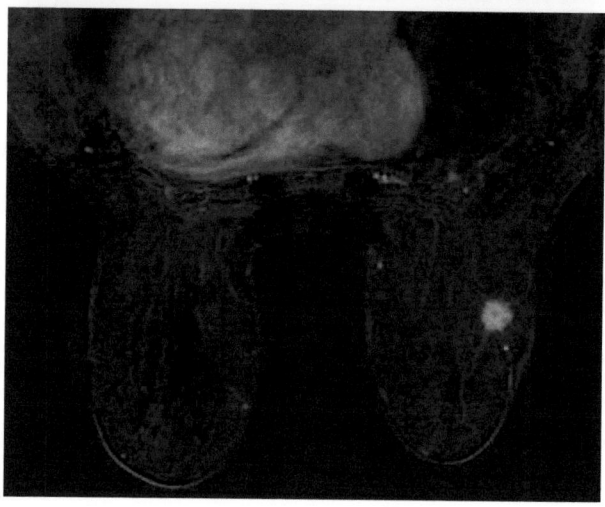

Fig. 1: Contrast-enhanced sequences.

a) T1-weighted sequence performed in the 2nd minute after administration of contrast medium.

b) Contrast-enhanced T1-weighted sequence subtracted in the 2nd minute.

The signal registered during passage of the contrast medium bolus is used to generate the so-called time/intensity curves (TICs) which reflect the absorption in the tissues. This signal evidences different enhancement values on the images. There are three main types of TICs:

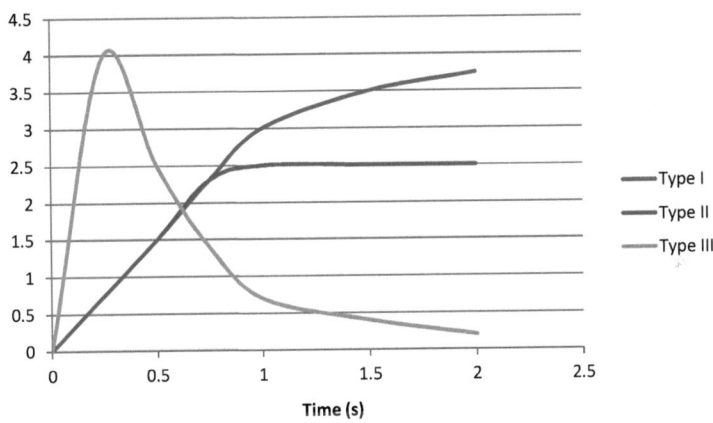

Fig. 2: TICs

- *Type I is characterized by slow, progressive wash-in and wash-out. This pattern indicates benign lesions with poor vascularization and therefore slow proliferation.*

- *Type II is characterized by slow wash-in followed by a plateau meaning slow, gradual and persistent impregnation with contrast medium. This pattern is typical of borderline lesions and requires further investigation using additional sequences and morphological evaluation of the lesion.*

- *Type III is characterized by rapid wash-in with a sudden rise followed by an early and steep wash-out. This is typical of lesions with intense vascularity and uncontrolled growth suggesting malignancy.*

Analysis of the TICs provides information on the physiopathological properties of the tissues, such as blood flow, vascular permeability, angiogenesis and volume of the vascularized tissues.

To obtain the MRI sequences, a ROI is chosen and the images are acquired autonomously on the basis of the arrival of contrast medium in the ROI, i.e. a few seconds before, during and after intravenous injection of contrast medium. Each image corresponds to one time instant and each pixel of each sequence of images generates a curve of intensity values. Signal variations correlate with the concentration of contrast medium in the tissues, and each instant after bolus injection therefore depends on the vascularization, vascular permeability, neoangiogenesis, etc. These data permit generation of a specific map of the microvascularization.

MRI is particularly sensitive also to low concentrations of paramagnetic contrast medium present in the tissues, and image acquisition is based on two different physiochemical properties[5]:

- **Relaxation time:** the presence of contrast medium reduces T1 and T2 relaxation times; this ability is used to generate a positive enhancement on T1-weighted images;

- **Magnetic susceptibility effects:** when paramagnetic contrast medium reaches the vessels of a tissue, and the magnetic susceptibility of the contrast medium is greater than that of the fluid which is already present in the tissue, an area of magnetic inhomogeneity is created between the intra- and extravascular surfaces. This inhomogeneity yields negative enhancement on T2-weighted images.

This means that the obtained images allow an immediate evaluation of the vascular pattern and at the same time a tentative qualitative evaluation of the examined tissue.

The distribution of contrast medium allows distinction of different vascular patterns. A homogeneous pattern is characteristic of benign lesions, whereas a heterogeneous pattern is characteristic of both borderline and malignant lesions. Sometimes, this pattern is ambiguous or there is a rim enhancement pattern which is characteristic of malignant lesions with elevated mitotic activity, rapid growth and central necrosis due to lack of angiogenesis, which is greater in the peripheral area of the lesion.

However, also a quantitative analysis is achieved thanks to technological progress and increasingly rapid sequences, with full breast coverage in a few seconds. The passage of contrast agent through the vascular bed is registered as the volume transfer constant (Ktrans), a parameter providing a quantitative measure of qualitative modifications, e.g. increased vascular permeability which is a surrogate measure of tumor angiogenesis[6]. Benign and malignant breast lesions are differentiated on the basis of microvascular features revealed by the different distribution of contrast medium and therefore by the pharmacokinetic curves, which depict the time/intensity rate.

Dynamic contrast-enhanced MRI (DCE-MRI) sequences are considered the gold standard for characterizing breast lesions[19]. However, this examination requires integration with pre-contrast T2-weighted sequences as well as DWI sequences and ADC map. Pre-contrast T2-weighted sequences provide a morphological evaluation of the lesion and the definition of margins, which may be spiculated, irregular, regular or lobulated, in descending order of malignancy, while DWI and ADC map can improve diagnostic sensitivity and post-operative management.

3. DWI sequences and ADC map

One of the more recent MRI applications provides the possibility to measure *in vivo* the mean diffusion time of water molecules in biological tissues. Diffusion time is thus one of three flow signal parameters in addition to perfusion and macroscopic blood flow.

The random motion of water molecules is linked to the thermal energy of the particles and the impact with neighboring molecules. This motion is also referred to as the Brownian motion, and it gives origin to the diffusion phenomena.

In order to sensitize the MRI sequences to the diffusion, two gradient pulses of opposite sign but of equal intensity and duration, are used instead of a single long pulse divided by a time interval. The spins of the water molecules depend on their position when the first gradient is added, and on their position after the interval, i.e. when the second gradient is added. As this movement is random in the Brownian motion, the spins of the different molecules present different phase variations with loss of phase coherence and signal. This loss of signal is caused entirely by the diffusion of the molecules and is described by the following equation:

$$S = S_0 \, e^{-bADC}$$

where S and S_0 are the respective signal intensities of diffusion with and without diffusion sensitization. ADC is the apparent diffusion coefficient, which varies according to the type of fluid and the temperature. ADC describes the area covered by a molecule in stochastic motion over a unit of time, and it is defined as "apparent", because it does in fact not take into account some substantial aspects, such as the proportion of water molecules which is linked to the macromolecules and the direction of the structures, such as cell membranes and organelles; b is the degree of sensitization, i.e. of "weighing", at the diffusion of the sequence. The higher the value of b, the higher is diffusion sensitization.

15

The loss of signal therefore depends exponentially on the diffusion: low diffusion of water molecules is characteristic of highly cellular tissues and corresponds to a low signal loss; vice versa, in high diffusion tissue, the molecules are free to move and cause a high signal loss.

For this reason it is possible to calculate ADC maps on the basis of at least two DWIs with different b-values, e.g. 0 and 1000 s/mm^2. These maps are not only significant from a qualitative point of view, but they are genuine quantitative maps in which the signal intensity of each voxel is at the same time the mean value of that voxel[7] (Fig. 3).

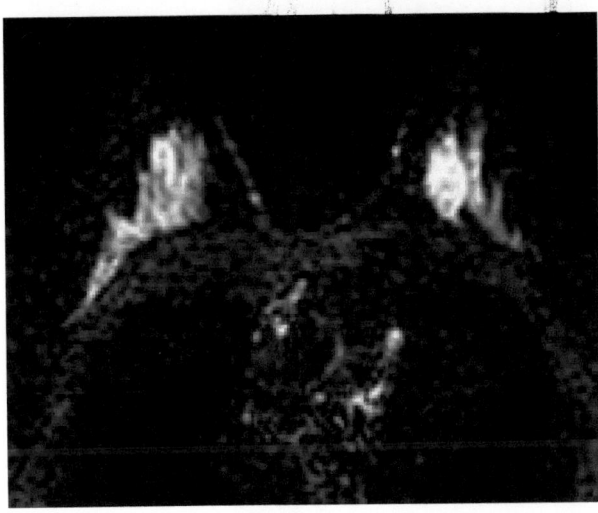

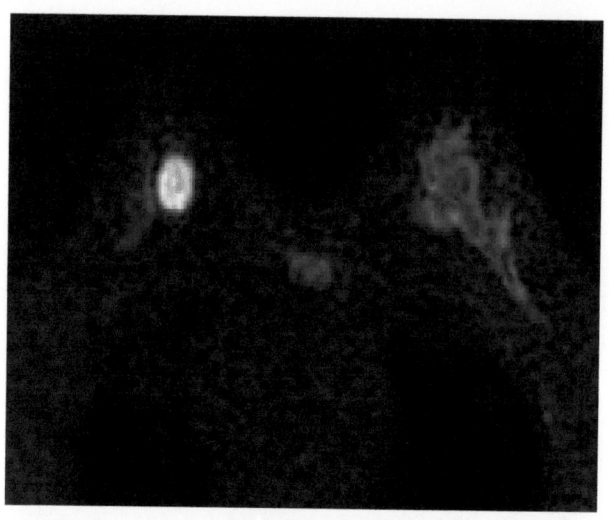

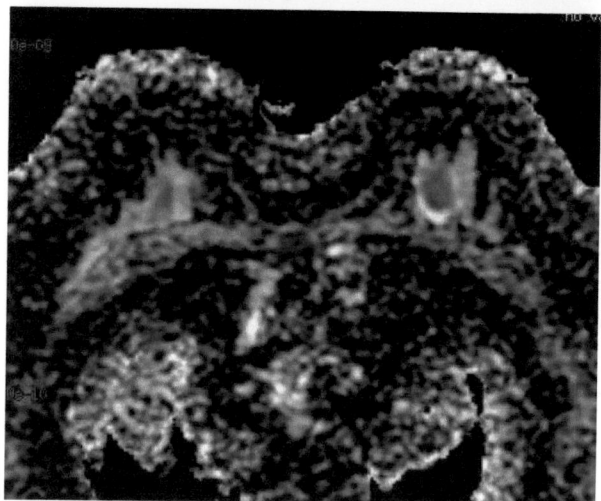

Fig. 3: Invasive ductal carcinoma of the left breast: DWI sequences and ADC map

map

  a) *DWI sequence using b-value =0*

  b) *DWI sequence using b-value = 1000*

  c) *ADC map*

DWI was initially introduced for the assessment of ischemic areas of the brain[21]. Later this technique was further developed for application in other fields, such as the breast. In breast diseases, DWI is used for differentiating between benign and malignant lesions, as the ADC map provides a noninvasive classification of malignancy by suggesting the histological nature of the lesion, thus increasing sensitivity of MRI.

4. Advantages, limitations and contraindications to MRI

4.1 Advantages

MRI has rapidly spread to many fields of oncologic imaging thanks to the elevated diagnostic accuracy and also to a series of advantages over older techniques such as US, CT and plain film radiology (RX). The advantages of MRI are:

- Possibility to acquire images without the use of ionizing radiation (X-rays) unlike CT and RX, thus permitting repeated scanning;

- Images can be acquired in multiple planes (axial, sagittal, coronal, oblique), without repositioning the patient (CT imaging has only recently acquired the ability to reconstruct the images in multiple planes with the same spatial resolution);

- MRI delivers better soft-tissue contrast than CT and RX and is therefore the most adequate examination for assessing organs such as the brain, spine, joints and breast;

- Thanks to the possibility to select a signal weighting which is adequate for the tissue under investigation, angiographic images can be obtained without the use of contrast medium (unlike CT and conventional angiography);

- Advanced techniques such as DWI, spectroscopic and perfusion MRI provide specific tissue characterization, thereby adding functional information to the acquisition of macroscopic images.

4.2 Disadvantages

There are some disadvantages and difficulties linked to MRI scanning.

MRI is more expensive than CT, and the longer duration of image acquisition impacts patient comfort. The images are furthermore easily impaired by artifacts, which must be recognized and reduced or eliminated.

MRI scanning is not safe in patients with certain types of metal implants/foreign objects, and specific safety measures are required to prevent severe injury to patients and staff. This requires special MRI safe equipment and strict adherence to MRI safety protocols.

4.3 3.0 Tesla

The most widely used magnets are 1.5 Tesla (1.5T), but also stronger magnets are increasingly being used in breast MRI. Particularly, magnets with a 3.0 Tesla (3.0T) magnetic field are now commonly employed in clinical practice. The power of the magnetic field affects some features of the produced image, such as the signal-to-noise ratio (SNR), spatial resolution and acquisition time[22-25]. It is therefore important to understand the possible advantages and disadvantages of 3.0T MRI in order to compare the performance with that of a 1.5T MRI scanner.

A magnetic field with high intensity produces a proportional increase in SNR with improved spatial and temporal resolution. The increased spectral separation of fat and water in 3.0T images allows for better fat suppression that improves visualization of breast lesions. On the other hand, the technical quality of a 3.0T image is challenged by the lack of homogeneity due to higher B_0 and B_1 fields, and thus by a greater incidence of magnetic susceptibility artifacts. However, these potential disadvantages can be overcome by adjusting the imaging parameters, such as repetition time (RT), echo time (ET) and flip angle.

The main differences between high-field and low-field magnets are:

a) Increased SNR

b) Increased spatial resolution

c) Increased temporal resolution

d) Increased specific absorption rate (SAR)

e) Increased acoustic noise

a) Signal to noise ratio (SNR)

SNR is defined as follows:

$$SNR = \frac{i_m}{\sigma i}$$

where i_m is the mean value of the image in a certain area and σi is the relative standard deviation.

SNR is measured by calculating the difference in signal intensity between the ROI and the background (usually chosen from the air surrounding the object). In air, all signals are noise. The difference between signal and background noise is separated by the standard deviation of the signal from the background, which is an indicator of the variability of the background.

SNR is proportional to the volume of the voxel and to the square root of the number or averages and phase steps (assuming constant voxel size). Since averaging and increasing the phase steps take time, SNR is closely related to the acquisition time.

In MRI, the SNR can be improved by:

- using spin echo sequences instead of gradient echo sequences;
- decreasing noise values using signal average: the images are registered and the average is calculated. The signals are present in each average image so that their contribution to the resulting image is additive. The increased SNR resulting from the average signal is proportional to the square root of the number of averaged images,

commonly referred to as the number of excitations (Nex) or number of detections (see below);

-   increasing the signal by decreasing ET and increasing RT.

SNR can furthermore be improved by changing the scan parameters. Assuming that all other factors remain the same, SNR can be improved by:

-   decreasing matrix size
-   increasing field of view (FOV)
-   increasing slice thickness
-   increasing number of excitations (Nex) which is an indicator of how many times each line of the area under investigation is acquired during the scanning. In order to obtain a sufficiently accurate sample signal, the MRI software permits more than one radiofrequency (RF) transmission and reception of the same number of signals for each sector of the matrix. The average of the obtained values provides a sample signal whose accuracy is directly proportional to the number of excitations: by doubling the number of measurements also acquisition time is doubled.

NEX	MATRIX	FOV	THICKN ESS	SNR
↑	↓	↑	↑	↑

Table 1: *SNR variations*

In theory, the signal increases proportionally to the square of the value of the magnetic field intensity, and the noise increases linearly. This implies that in an ideal SNR of a 3.0T system, the signal would be nearly twice as good as that of a 1.5T system. However, the actual improvement is only 30%-60%, due to the increased susceptibility to artifacts in many tissues. If SNR is increased, spatial resolution and/or acquisition time can be improved depending on which of the two is more important in the specific case.

b) *Spatial resolution*

Spatial resolution is the smallest possible measurable size variation of the method, i.e. the value of the last figure obtained in the measurement. In practice, spatial resolution describes the ability to distinguish between two closely located points, such as in a system of alternate black and white bars the spatial resolution is thus the ability to distinguish between them and it is expressed as the frequency domain in line pairs per millimeter (lp/mm).

In an imaging system, the spatial resolution is the maximum number of line pairs per unit of distance that can be counted correctly. If f_{max} is the resolution of a system, $h_{min} = \frac{1}{2\,f_{max}}$ corrisponds to the size of the smallest structure that can be distinguished. However, it should be kept in mind that the selected interaction generally sets an intrinsic limit of the MRI detector to the resolution which must be considered.

In MRI, spatial resolution is defined also by the size of the imaging voxels , i.e. the volumetric elements that constitute the body under analysis and correspond to the two-dimensional pixels of the produced image. We can imagine the voxels as rectangular solids with three dimensions, and the resolution is often different in the three directions. However, the dimension of the voxel, and therefore the spatial resolution, depends on the size of the matrix, FOV, and slice thickness.

The **matrix** is a group of small equal-sized areas (pixels) arranged in rows (horizontal) and columns (vertical). It is characterized by the number of pixels and can be symmetric, e.g. 128 x 128 or 256 x 256, or asymmetric, e.g. 512 x 256 or 256 x 192, etc.

A matrix measuring 256 x 256 requires a longer acquisition time, because more rows and more columns must be filled, but it gives a better spatial resolution as the pixels are smaller. A matrix measuring 128 x 128 requires a shorter acquisition time and allows up to four times increase in signal intensity thanks to an increased number of protons resonating within the voxel.

The matrix dimension is the number of frequency encoding steps (MatrFreq) in one direction, and the number of phase encoding steps (MatrPh) in the direction opposed to that of the image plane (Fig. 4). These values may be different, but MatrPh is usually lower than or equal to MatrFreq.

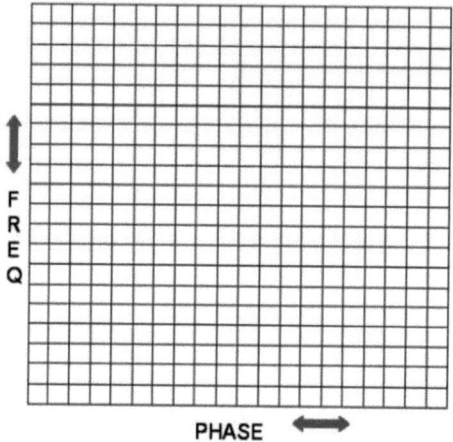

Fig. 4: *Matrix*

If all other parameters are kept constant, increase in the number of frequency encoding steps or the number of phase encoding steps will generate an increase in resolution as well as a variation in the other parameters, as shown in the following tables (Tables 1 and 2).

MAT FREQ	TIME	RESOLUTION	SNR	SLICES
↑	=	↑	↓	↓=

Table 2: *Variation in the matrix: frequency encoding steps*

23

MAT PHASE	TEMPO	RISOLUZIONE	SNR	N° STRATI
↑	↑	↑	↓	=

Table 3: *Variation in the matrix: phase encoding steps*

Frequency encoding depends on the speed of the RF signal which is transmitted and sampled by the scanner. An increase in the encoding values of the sampling frequency causes no increase in acquisition time, whereas an increase in the number of phase encoding steps will proportionally increase image acquisition time. This is the reason why images with a lower number of phase encoding steps than frequency encoding steps are used, e.g. 128x256 or 192x256.

FOV (field of view) is the size of the area that the frequency matrix and phase encoding matrix express. The relationship between FOV and the matrix size indicates the size of the voxels in the plane. Therefore, an increase in FOV in both directions increases the size of the voxels and decreases the resolution; conversely, a decrease in FOV improves the spatial resolution (Table 4).

MAT FREQ	MAT PHASE	FOV	RESOLUTION
↑	↑	↓	↑

Table 4: *Variation in spatial resolution resulting from variations in FOV and matrix.*

The depth is the third dimension of the voxel; it is determined by the slice thickness which is nearly always the largest dimension of the voxels in 3D images. It is thus understandable that the resolution which is perpendicular to the image plane is the lowest. This is linked to the maximum resistance of the gradient coils in axis z and to the time limits that determine the number of sections available.

A problem linked to the use of an asymmetric voxel is that it may cause considerable partial-volume artifacts affecting the longest side (usually in the direction of MatrPh). For example:

- FOV 240mm, MatrFreq 320 and MatrPh 320 result in a square pixel of 0.67 mm x 0.67 mm ($0.44mm^2$ surface);

- FOV 240mm, MatrFreq 512 and MatrPh 256 result in a rectangular pixel of 0.47 mm x 0.94 mm ($0.44mm^2$ surface).

In these two cases, the resolution is the same (linked to the area of the pixels) but the acquired image is of a higher quality when a symmetric matrix 320x320 is used.

Slice thickness is the thickness of the part of the body which is visible in that particular layer. In fact, the image that is produced is the representation of a volumetric three-dimensional body. This means that the pixel displayed in an MRI image represents a volume (voxel) in which two dimensions are related to the pixels and the third to the thickness.

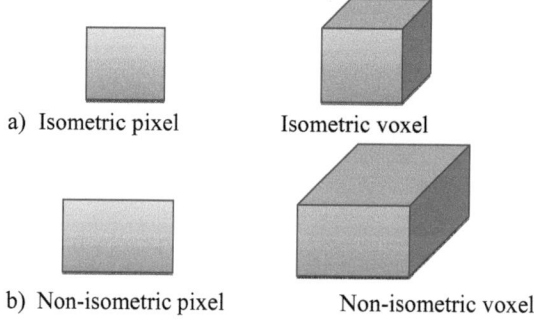

a) Isometric pixel   Isometric voxel

b) Non-isometric pixel   Non-isometric voxel

Fig. 5: *Isometric and non-isometric pixels and voxels.*

Pixels with two identical dimensions simplify the production and particularly the interpretation of the voxels, which are defined as isometric (Fig. 5a). However in standard images, the reader usually has to work with voxels in which the two dimensions of the pixels are considerably shorter than that of the thickness, and they are defined as non-isometric voxels (Fig. 5b).

Because each voxel is shown in only one gray scale value, all tissues present in its volume are considered as a single structure, even if several different signals are coexisting. If, for example, the voxel volume contains both isointense and hypointense tissues, the voxel will appear isointense.

The thinner the slices the more detailed information is contained in the voxel, and more singular features of the examined tissues are obtained. Basically, a reduced slice thickness should always be preferred, but this choice creates considerable technical problems.

- If slice thickness is reduced, SNR decreases with loss of image quality and Nex must be increased to recover lost signals resulting in prolonged acquisition time;
- If the number of slices remains the same, the study will be reduced to a smaller part of the body;
- In order to study the same anatomic site, the number of slices must be increased resulting in prolonged acquisition time.

The choice of slice thickness therefore depends on the anatomical structure of interest and is entirely linked to partial-volume artifact. There are protocols providing the use of increased slice thickness in order to exploit partial-volume artifact mainly in sequences exploiting a high intrinsic contrast between the tissues.

c) Temporal resolution

Temporal resolution is the period of time required for the acquisition of a single frame of the dynamic process, i.e. the imaging speed.

The concept of temporal resolution is fundamental to cardiac CT and MRI in which a rapidly beating heart is imaged over the order of milliseconds into multiple frame-captures. In MRI, the time gap between consecutive images indicates the temporal resolution which is given by the formula:

Temporal resolution = VPS x RT

Where VPS = views per segment, a user-defined variable, and RT = repetition time. If TR is 10ms and there are 5 views per segment, the temporal resolution will be 50ms.

d) Specific absorption rate (SAR)

SAR is defined as the RF power (joule) deposited in the tissues (kg). The upper limit established by the Food and Drug Administration (FDA) is a quantity which causes a temperature increase by 1 centigrade in any tissue [http://www.fda.gov/]. SAR is proportional to the square of the static magnetic field strength (B_0), meaning that a 3.0T system is four times more powerful than a 1.5T system. SAR is furthermore proportional to the

- duration of the RF pulse
- number of pulses
- slice number
- flip angle

In standard spin echo sequences, flip angle exceeds 90 degrees with a consequent increase in magnetic energy. As a result, there is an increased use of gradient echo sequences.

e) Acoustic noise

The rapid alteration of currents within the gradient coils of a high-field magnet produces various types of acoustic noise, and adequate protection measures are therefore required within the MRI unit and in the examination room.

Thanks to the increase in SNR as well as spatial and temporal resolution, 3.0T MRI is a more accurate imaging technique owing to its diagnostic accuracy in breast cancer and other pathologies. Several studies have reported a higher image quality and diagnostic confidence obtained with 3.0T MRI as well as improved characterization of the lesions. This includes a better definition of lobulated and spiculated margins, which would otherwise have appeared regular, improved detection of occult cancer, and detection of a greater number of occult malignant foci leading to the diagnosis of multifocal, multicentric and/or bilateral breast cancer[8]. However, there are still few reports in the literature on breast MRI using 3.0T.

4.4 Artifacts

A variety of artifacts may be encountered in MRI images, directly proportional to the strength of the magnetic field. It is very important to be able to recognize imaging artifacts to avoid misinterpretation, but it is also essential to know what can be done to prevent them from being generated, if possible.

MRI artifacts are caused by a distribution of signals that do not correspond to the parameters of the studied tissues[20]. The main component contributing to the generation of artifacts is the encoding, and the artifacts are therefore classified according to the encoding:

- Artifacts in the direction of:
  - Phase:
    a) Aliasing
    b) Radiofrequency
    c) Movement
  - Frequency
    d) Chemical shift
  - Phase and frequency
    e) Gibbs or truncation artifacts
    f) Slice

g) Multislice crosstalk

- Artifacts independent of the direction of phase-encoding or frequency-encoding linked to:
  - Signal
    - h) Magnetic susceptibility
    - i) Inhomogeneous static magnetic field (SMF)

a. **Aliasing artifacts** are the reflection of the organs and tissues located outside the FOV image. It occurs when the FOV in the phase-encoding direction is smaller than the body-part being imaged and particularly in the study of the abdomen, whereas it is rare in the study of the breast. Nevertheless, it can be avoided in various ways:

- Inverting the phase-encoding direction, which must be oriented along the short axis of the body-part being examined;
- Increasing FOV; however as previously pointed out, this involves reduction of the spatial resolution;
- Increasing matrix size in the phase-encoding direction thereby doubling FOV in that direction;
- Saturating the regions located outside FOV.

The last two options are automatically selected by the MRI scanner: the first in case of an even number of acquisitions, the second in case of an odd number of acquisitions.

b. **RF artifacts** cross the image in the presence of one or more bands joined in the phase-encoding direction. They are caused by interference of RF waves coming from the monitor, neon lamps or other equipment using the same RF amplitude as the impulse used in the scanning, but they can also be caused by electrostatic discharges from electrical machines. Normally, RF signals are prevented from being added to the data collected from the patient by the presence of the Faraday cage. A similar type of artifact is the *feed-through* artifact, where the interference comes from the MRI scanner itself and not from the environment and in the presence of only one band. It affects only one pixel and crosses through the center of the image. This artifact is more common in T2-weighted sequences with fat saturation. **Motion artifacts** are the most frequent causes of image degradation. They may be voluntary or not, caused by the flow of liquids, respiratory movements or heart breath. In the frequency-encoding direction, data are obtained in a few milliseconds, while data are collected during the entire scanning in the phase-encoding direction. The acquired data will therefore be placed in the wrong pixel in the final image. The artifacts are presented in various ways: band, ring or ghost images. Possible solutions are:

- Increase the number of acquisitions; this solution is used particularly in abdominal imaging;

- Selection of the phase-encoding direction; this solution is used particularly in breast imaging;

- Flow compensation: pulse sequences include blood flow compensation, unless it is turbulent;

- Cardiac gating in heart imaging by synchronizing the imaging sequences with an electrocardiogram;

- Phase-encoding orientation;

- Scans performed with the patient holding his breath, reducing the acquisition time to 10-20 seconds; this method is possible only in patients who collaborate;

- Presaturation pulse applied to a selected region to eliminate the signal from that region.

c. **Chemical shift** appears as a white band and black interface between two different tissues with different properties. This artifact frequently occurs at the interface between abundant tissues such as mammary fat and mammary gland and it occurs because fat proton resonance frequency is slower than that of other protons, such as water protons. Both groups of protons are excited upon the arrival of RF-pulses and fat protons as well as water protons get in resonance, but with different

30

frequencies. As frequency encoding is used to determine the position of the hydrogen atoms in the image, the frequency variation caused by the chemical shift is converted into a displacement (shift) of the position along the readout gradient. From here the fat proton image is shifted in the frequency encoding direction compared to the water proton image. This shift is proportional to the intensity of the magnetic field and the readout gradient; the latter is the only parameter which can be modified.

d. **Truncation** is also called Gibbs artifact. Is consists of alternating light and dark bands and occurs in regions with high contrast, e.g. between muscle and fat. It occurs in both directions, the phase encoding direction and the frequency encoding direction, and it is most evident in the phase encoding direction in the presence of rectangular matrices. This artifact is more pronounced in low matrices as the Fourier transform is discrete.

e. **Multislice crosstalk** occurs because the intensity pattern varies between adjacent layers, if layers with high intensity alternate with layers with low intensity. This phenomenon is caused by the acquisition of even layered images before odd layered images. The alternation appears as a partial overlapping of layers which have already been acquired. The solution to this problem is to increase the gap between the layers, generally up to 10%, but it can be increased up to 25% in sequences which are particularly susceptible to these artifacts, such as inversion recovery.

f. **Magnetic susceptibility** is the reduction of the signal intensity at the interface between two adjacent tissues and it appears as gradient echo and turbo gradient echo sequences in regions such as air/bone tissue interfaces.

g. **Inhomogeneous static magnetic field** is caused by the presence of metal structures (clips, dentures, orthopedic implants, etc.). The image shows a black or dark area with no signal surrounded by an asymmetric band with intense signal. This artifact is particularly evident on T2-weighted scans and particularly in gradient echo sequences.

4.5 Controindications and limitations

Unlike other imaging modalities, such as mammography and CT, MRI does not use ionizing radiation, but biological risk to the patient is not completely excluded. There is in fact a possibility that the magnetic field and the emitted pulsed RF waves may interact with molecules and organs containing ferromagnetic, paramagnetic or diamagnetic materials.

The MRI scanner behaves like a large magnet with a strong static magnetic field that attracts ferrous material. When exposed to such a magnetic force, metal objects in the body may behave like projectiles moving towards the magnet. The presence of metal objects is therefore an obvious contraindication to MRI scanning.

Contraindications are classified as follows:

Absolute contraindications:

- Presence of a pace maker which is not MRI-safe;

- Presence of ferrous metal objects, Cochlear implants or prosthetic contact lenses;

- Body weight exceeding 130 kg;

- Pregnancy is not an absolute contraindication; however, in the absence of randomized clinical trials reported in the literature assessing the effects of MRI on the fetus, a possible scanning should be carried out only in agreement with the patient's general physician.

Relative contraindications:

- Presence of coronary artery or ureteral stents up to six weeks after implantation, except those made of titanium. Stents positioned before 1995 must be certified as MRI-safe;

- Presence of metallic implants, clips, except those made of titanium, heart valves, spine implants, neurostimulators and implanted drug infusion pumps unless they are certified as MRI-safe;

- Fixed dentures, which may degrade the image quality due to metal artifacts;

- Tattoos which can deteriorate or cause metal artifacts;

- Claustrophobia, as claustrophobic reactions may prevent the scanning procedure from being completed; this condition therefore requires special attention.

In case of contrast enhanced MRI, more safety precautions are required. Paramagnetic contrast medium is better tolerated than iodinated contrast media owing to the smaller volume and reduced number of moles of substance which do not involve risk of toxicity. The main drawback concerns patients with pre-existing reaction to paramagnetic contrast medium, but this adverse event is very rare. However, a small number of patients have developed a hitherto unknown disease, nephrogenic systemic fibrosis (NSF). It is caused by accumulation of gadolinium-based contrast medium and occurs in patients with severe renal impairment and/or patients who have undergone liver transplantation. This disease is obviously an absolute contraindication to the use of contrast medium.

5. Breast carcinoma: prognostic factors

Since 1990, breast cancer death rate has decreased by 1%-2% per year in most European countries thanks to early detection and to a more efficient treatment[27]. Breast cancer is a complex and costly disease, which requires management by a well functioning team of health care operators, as a multidisciplinary approach has proved to reduce mortality rate and improve the patients' quality of life.

Diagnosis and management of breast cancer requires a specific procedure as stipulated by EUSOMA in 2010; a total of 17 steps, divided into 4 groups:

Diagnosis:

1. Initial diagnosis through physical breast examination and conventional imaging techniques, such as US and mammography to allow proper diagnostic assessment and to identify size, site and possible multifocal and/or contralateral disease.

2. Further assessment to establish the malignant or benign nature of the lesion through fine needle aspiration and/or core biopsy;

3. Presurgical diagnosis in women with confirmed breast carcinoma, in sito or invasive (C5 or B5);

4. Evaluation of predictive and prognostic factors as recommended by EUSOMA:

   - Histological type
   - Grading (according to the EU guidelines)
   - Hormone receptor status: ER and PgR

The first two points seem to be very important, as they may influence prognosis and also predict development of multifocal lesions and distant metastases.

   - HER2 status
   - Pathological stage (T and N)
   - Size in mm
   - Perivascular invasion
   - Distance to nearest radial margin

5. Waiting time, i.e. time between the date of first diagnostic examination within the breast unit and the date of surgery or start of other treatment.

6. Access to preoperative MRI scanning

7. Access to genetic counseling, necessary but not mandatory

Therapy: surgery and loco-regional treatment

8. The clinical case is submitted to the attention of a multidisciplinary team to decide on the best treatment for the type of cancer and the general condition of the patient in question.

34

9. Surgical approach: lumpectomy, quadrantectomy or mastectomy with or without lymphadenectomy (lymph node-negative biopsy or sentinel node biopsy), lymph node sampling or total lymphadenectomy.

10. Post-operative radiotherapy which decreases local recurrence risk and increases long-term survival.

11. Avoid surgical over-treatment, thereby encouraging the patient to accept treatment, improve postoperative radiation therapy performance to allow better aesthetic results.

Therapy: systemic treatment

12. Appropriate hormone therapy should be offered to patients with endocrine sensitive breast cancer. However, the last St. Gallen consensus paper pointed out a particular receptor combination: ER-negative/PgR-positive tumors; this receptor structure is probably artifactual. Patients with ER-negative and PgR-positive breast cancer can therefore not be treated with hormone therapy[28].

13. Appropriate adjuvant chemotherapy or other medical therapy should be offered to patients with invasive tumors which are endocrine insensitive or ER-negative (T>1 cm or N +). Invasive HER2-positive carcinomas (IHC 3+ or FISH+) should be treated with specific monoclonal antibody drugs, Trastuzumab combined with chemotherapy. In contrast, inflammatory carcinoma or hormone-negative locally advanced breast tumors, which are unresectable, should be treated with adjuvant chemotherapy.

Post-treatment: staging, maintenance, follow-up and rehabilitation

14. Appropriate staging should include US of the liver, chest RX and skeletal scintigraphy. CT, skeletal RX, MRI and PET can be performed when recommended by the clinicians.

15. An adequate follow-up should be planned. Asymptomatic patients should undergo routine mammography on an annual basis and clinical evaluation every 6 months in the first 5 years after the operation.

16. Excessive and inappropriate follow-up more than local assessment should be avoided, as randomized trials have reported no survival benefit from intensive screening for asymptomatic metastatic disease.

17. Specialized nurse counseling should be available to provide patients undergoing treatment with information and support.

As the therapy is tailored to the individual patient, TNM classification based on size (T), lymph node status (N) and distant metastases (M) at diagnosis is nowadays supported and partly substituted in the therapeutic planning by prognostic factors. The variability of these factors has been assessed in groups of clinically and anatomopathologically homogeneous patients, and the use has led to a more accurate biological characterization of the lesions in each individual patient.

Particularly, two aspects are considered: morphology and biological function.

- Assessment of morphology includes the following characterizing features:
    - Histotype, i.e. differentiation of cancer cell type, such as ductal, lobular, mucinous, papillary, and tubular carcinoma, and classification as tumor in situ, tumor not breaking through the basement membrane and invasive or infiltrating tumor;
    - Grading, classified 1, 2 or 3 on the basis of characteristics such as mitotic count, the presence of tubular formations and the degree of atypia;
    - Nuclear grade, classified 1, 2 or 3 according to shape, atypia and coloring of the nucleus in the tumor cells;

    Histotype, grading and nuclear grade form the expression of cell differentiation and therefore of intrinsic tumor aggressiveness.
    - Lymphatic vessel invasion, which is defined by the presence of neoplastic emboli within the peritumoral lymphatic vessels;
    - Angiogenesis owing to endothelial angiogenic growth factor production with greater proliferative capacity and metastatic spread.

36

Embolization along the lymph channels and angiogenesis demonstrate the tumor's ability to invade other tissues and therefore to set metastases.

- The biofunctional aspect includes prognostic factors which were previously derived from cell biology and more recently from molecular biology:

   ▪ Estrogen (ER) and progesterone (PgR) receptors are steroid hormone receptors expressing cell differentiation. The new guidelines issued by the American Society of Clinical Oncology (ASCO) for immunohistochemical testing consider tumors positive if at least 30% of the cells are ER- and PgR-positive29. These receptors are taken into consideration in the prognosis, but particularly in the therapeutic management. PgR expression is linked to a molecular transduction cascade where estradiol binds to the estrogen receptor-alpha. The activity of these two receptors is so closely connected that William et al30 defined the presence/absence of ER only as an independent prognostic factor. According to this study, ER-negative tumors are more likely to develop metastases, and 5-year survival rate is reduced. The presence of ER and PgR is thus a positive prognostic factor, and luckily this receptor structure is present in over 70% of breast cancers. It is a sign of a high degree of cell differentiation, and this becomes the target of therapeutic drugs such as tamoxifen, used in combination with chemotherapy in women before and after menopause. In premenopausal patients with ER-positive tumors, tamoxifen has proved to reduce the risk of recurrence and death, particularly when combined with chemotherapy. In contrast, tamoxifen is not significantly effective in premenopausal patients with ER-negative tumors. In postmenopausal patients, tamoxifen reduces the risk of recurrence and death, also in patients with ER-negative tumors, but this drug is more effective in patients with ER-positive tumors.

   ▪ Proliferative activity allows assessment of various phases of the cell division cycle. It is thus possible to quantify the fraction of cells in the S phase, i.e. the phase of DNA synthesis, or the entire population of proliferating cells. In order to quantify the cells in the S phase, indicators

37

such as thymidine labelling index (TLI) or 5-bromo-2'-deoxyuridine labeling index (BrdU LI) can be used. This implies incorporation of thymidine or bromodeoxyuridine into the viable cells and subsequent evaluation with autoradiography, immunohistochemical testing or cytofluorometry. Also the S phase fraction can be quantified using cytofluorometry through assessment of nuclear DNA content using flow cytometry, quantified as standard cubic feet per minute (SCFM). On the other hand, assessment of the entire population of proliferating cells includes detection of enzymes, such as DNA polymerase and thymidine kinase, or antigens, such as Ki-67 and proliferating cell nuclear antigen (PCNA) which are linked to the proliferative process and therefore supposed to be present in all proliferating cells. Otherwise, detection of proteins bound to the nucleolus organizer regions (AgNORs) is required.

- TLI has been validated as a prognostic parameter in all studies owing to its biological and clinical significance. The principle of BrdU LI is similar to that of TLI, but reliability and reproducibility of BrdU LI are lower compared to TLI. The SCFM phase method is still being tested and its prognostic significance in breast cancer has still not been definitively confirmed. The results involving Ki-67 assessment with anti-Ki-67 antibody (MIB-1) seem to be adequately consolidated, whereas reports on PCNA and AgNORs are still too few.

- Ploidy implies quantification of the number of chromosomes using flow cytometry on fresh-frozen or formalin-fixed, paraffin-embedded samples to detect the nuclear DNA content and the presence of aneuploidy indicating the degree of cytological dedifferentiation.

- Invasiveness and metastatic potential is evidenced by the absence of cell adhesion proteins, such as E-cadherin, or protein expression, such as plasminogen activators, cathepsin D or other proteases.

- Expression of certain genes includes loss of tumor suppressor genes, mainly p53 protein, which is mutated in about 30% of breast cancers and the expression of proto-oncogenes and oncogenes which are important prognostic indicators correlating with disease recurrence (e.g. p53-mutated tumors are likely to relapse twice as frequently as tumors without p53-mutatation).

▪ HER2, also referred to as c-erbB2 or HER2-neu, belongs to the family of epithelial receptors and it is strongly associated with increased disease recurrence and a poor prognosis. Expression of HER2 protein is regulated by estrogen receptors, as estradiol regulates the HER2 expression. The presence of HER2 is assessed by measuring the expression of HER2 genes within the cancer cells or of HER2 molecules on the cell surface that will be higher than normal. Mainly two types of tests are used:

- HER2 fluorescence in-situ hybridization (FISH) is a diagnostic test for the detection of HER2 gene amplification in the tumor cell population and therefore of the overexpression of this molecule. The test result is expressed as 0+, 1+, 2+ or 3+.

- HER2 immunohistochemistry (IHC) is a diagnostic test for the detection of HER2 protein overexpression in the tumor cell population as a result of an increase in gene copy number. The test result is reported as a percentage.

About 35% of breast cancers develop in parallel with the HER2-neu gene amplification and protein overexpression. This receptor therefore becomes a therapeutic target in the adjuvant chemotherapy using the monoclonal antibody trastuzumab (Herceptin®) in combination with drugs such as doxorubicin, cyclophosphamide and a taxane (paclitaxel or docetaxel), or as a unimodal treatment after anthracycline based therapy.

▪ Bcl-2 is a proto-oncogene whose expression prevents programmed cell death or apoptosis. The absence of this expression is an important adverse prognostic factor, but its role is not independent of that of p53 with which it is significantly and inversely correlated.

6. Grading

Greenough was the first to point out the importance of grading as an independent prognostic factor. In a study published in 1925, he argued that there was a close relationship between cell morphology and the degree of malignancy[9–11].

To date, the most common grading system recommended by various international corporations, such as the World Health Organization (WHO), the American Joint Committee on Cancer (AJCC), the European Union (EU) and the Royal College of Pathologists (UK RCPath) is the Nottingham grading system (NGS) which is the Elston-Ellis modification of the old Scarff-Bloom-Richardson system. The accuracy of NGS has been demonstrated in numerous studies and it is widely validated[33,34]. To calculate the Nottingham Prognostic Index (NPI), the grading is combined with two other prognostic factors: tumor size and lymph node infiltration.

Histological classification can take place according to two systems, which evaluate the growth pattern and the degree of cell differentiation to establish histological tumor type and histological grade. Most breast tumors (60%-75%) are not histotype-specific; they are referred to as invasive breast cancer of no special type (NST) and have a poor prognosis. Histological grading therefore acquires a significant role in the clinical management, especially as NGS evaluation of tumor behavior is simple, inexpensive and easily repeatable, requiring only correct hematoxylin and eosin staining. To obtain the most accurate results, the Nottingham/Tenovus study recommends analysis of tumor samples immediately after surgical excision also to minimize artifacts from autolysis. When a sample has been dyed it is treated with hematoxylin-eosin.

Tumor grading is based on the evaluation of three morphological features, each of which is assigned a score from 1 to 3 (Table 5).

Histological features	Score
Tubule formation	
Diffuse > 75% of the tumor area	1
Moderate: 10%-75% of the tumor area	2
Mild or absent: <10% of the tumor area	3
Nuclear pleomorphism	
Uniform nuclear cells, small with regular outlines	1
Cells larger than normal, moderate variability in size and shape	2
Marked variation in size and shape	3
Mitotic count	
0-9 mitoses/10 hpf	1
10-19 mitoses /10 hpf	2
≥20 mitoses /10 hpf	3

Table 5: NGS (Nottingham grading system).

Hpf = high power field

- **Tubule formation**: tubule formation is assessed over the whole tumor. It is characterized by the presence of bright areas devoid of cells. Adequate fixation reduces the possibility of confounding with bright areas caused by shrinkage artifact; if tubule formation is present in more than 75% of the sample, 1 point is assigned, in 10%-75% of the sample 2 points and in less than 10% 3 points.

- **Nuclear pleomorphism** is a quantitative and qualitative parameter. If the nuclei are small with little increase in size compared to normal breast epithelial cells, with regular outlines, uniform nuclear chromatin and little variation in size, the sample is assigned 1 point; if the nuclei are larger than normal with visible nuclei, open vesicular nuclei presenting with moderate variability in both size and shape, the sample is assigned 2 points; if the nuclei present elevated variability in size and

41

shape, occasionally with very large and bizarre forms, prominent vesicles and often numerous nuclei, 3 points are assigned.

- **Mitotic count:** mitotic activity is most accurately evaluated using a minimum of 10x magnification in the peripheral area of the tumor where neoplastic growth is most active. The count includes only nuclei in visible metaphase, anaphase and telophase, whereas hyperchromatic and apoptotic nuclei are excluded. If there are up to 9 mitoses per 10x high-power field, the sample is assigned 1 point, from 10 to 19 mitosis per 10x high-power field 2 points, while a mitotic count equal to or greater than 20 per 10x high-power field is assigned 3 points.

- **Overall grade:** the points assigned to each category are added up to obtain a final score ranging from 3 to 9. Grades are assigned as follows (Fig. 6):
   o 3-5 points: grade 1 (G1), a well-differentiated tumor
   o 6-7 points: grade 2 (G2), a moderately differentiated tumor
   o 8-9 points: grade 3 (G3), a poorly differentiated or undifferentiated tumor

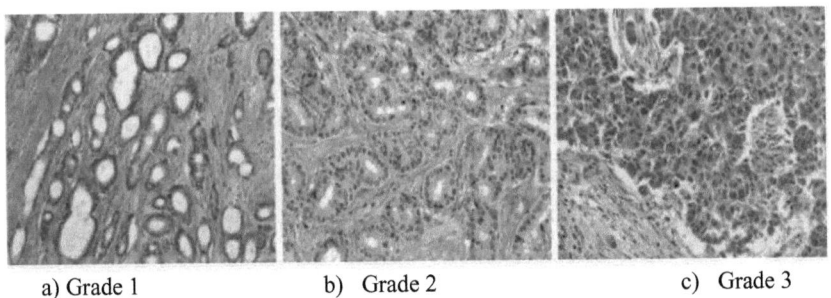

a) Grade 1   b) Grade 2   c) Grade 3

Fig. 6: Grade 1, 2 and 3:

a) Well-differentiated tumor (G1): elevated homology with the terminal duct lobular unit of normal breast tissue. There are abundant tubular formations in over 75% of the tumor tissue; an intermediate degree of nuclear pleomorphism and few mitoses.

b) Moderately differentiated tumor (G2): tubule formation in about 40% of the tumor, a moderate degree of nuclear pleomorphism and mitotic figures.

c) Poorly differentiated tumor (G3): a high degree of nuclear pleomorphism and numerous mitotic figures, absence of tubular formation (<10%).

42

However, according to some authors, grading has some limitations, such as the possibility that the obtained values are ambiguous, indeterminate and/or poorly reproducible, that they are borderline values which are equivocal (grade 2) like HER2 and Ki-67 expressions which may be borderline, intermediate or close to cut-off. These results may lead to doubts about tumor behavior and prevent the choice of a correct management.

This problem was overcome by the development of various prognostic indices (PIs), such as the Nottingham Prognostic Index (NPI) and Adjuvant! Online. The NPI was created in 1982 and uses a score that is obtained after evaluation of three parameters: tumor size, grading and lymph node involvement. The aim of Adjuvant! Online is to improve ten-year survival rate in patients with breast cancer, essentially on the basis of a positive or negative hormone-receptor status of the tumor.

Materials and methods

1. Patients

This retrospective study included revision of all breast mri examinations performed at the department of radiological sciences for local staging of breast cancer between april 2011 and January 2014.

Patients were enrolled in the study if the diagnostic procedure included the following:

- 3 Tesla MRI;
- Both DCE-MRI and DWI sequences;
- ADC value evaluation of the main lesion;
- Confirmation of MRI diagnosis by histopathological analysis after surgery or core biopsy;
- Histopathological diagnosis demonstrating invasive breast cancer;
- Histological analysis including molecular receptor assessment (ER, PgR; HER2) and Ki-67 index calculation.

Patients were excluded from the study if

- They had breast implants or expanders;
- Were undergoing follow-up after chemotherapy;
- Were receiving neo-adjuvant therapy;
- Images were not of a high diagnostic quality.

2. MRI scanning

All MRI scans were performed on a 3T magnet (Discovery 750; GE Healthcare, Milwaukee, WI, USA) using a dedicated eight-channel breast coil (8US TORSOPA) with the patient in the prone position. After localizer sequences taken in three orthogonal planes, the following sequences were acquired:

1) Axial T2-weighted single shot fast spin echo sequence using Dixon technique (IDEAL) for intravoxel fat-water separation (RT/ET 3500-5200/120-135 ms, matrix 352x224, FOV 370 x 370, NEX 1, slice thickness 3.5 mm);

2) Axial single shot fat suppressed echo-planar (EP) diffusion weighted sequence (RT/ET 2700/58 ms, matrix 100x120, FOV 360x360, NEX 6, slice thickness 5 mm) with diffusion-sensitizing gradient applied along the x, y, z axes and with a b-value of 0 and 1000 sec/mm^2;

3) Axial T1-weighted 3D dynamic gradient echo fat suppressed sequence (VIBRANT) (RT/ET 6.6/4.3 ms, flip angle 10°, matrix 512x256, NEX 1, slice thickness 2.4 mm), before and five times after intravenous contrast administration.

RT is the repetition time of the RF pulse, ET is echo time, FOV is the field of view, NEX the number of excitations and echo-planar DWI indicates the echo-planar diffusion-weighted sequence.

Contrast medium was Gadobenate Dimeglumine (Multihance®; Bracco Imaging, Milan, Italy) administered in a concentration of 0.2 mmol/kg injected through a 20 G intravenous cannula at the rate of 2 ml/sec using an automatic injector and followed by infusion of 15 ml saline solution at the same speed. Subtracted images were automatically derived from DCE-MRI.

Subtracted images were generated automatically by subtracting the mask from the images acquired after contrast administration. All technical details of the sequences are summarized in the following table:

Sequence	Value
T2 IDEAL axial	
RT/TE (ms)	3500-5200/120-135
Matrix	352 x 224
FOV (mm)	370 x 370

NEX	1
Slice thickness (mm)	3.5
T2 EP DWI axial	
RT/TE (ms)	2700/58
Matrix	100 x 120
FOV (mm)	360 x 360
NEX	6
B-values (s/mm2)	0-1000
Slice thickness (mm)	5
T1VIBRANT axial	
RT/TE (ms)	6.6/4.3
Angle	10°
FOV (mm)	380 x 380
Matrix	512 x 256
NEX	1
Slice thickness (mm)	2.4

Table 6: MRI parameters.

RT: Repetition time

ET: Echo time,

FOV: Field of view

NEX: Number of excitations

EP DWI: Echo-planar diffusion-weighted imaging

3. DWI sequences and analysis of ADC

After acquisition, the images were transferred to a workstation (Advantage Windows Workstation 4.4; GE Medical System, Milwaukee) for post-processing. For a quantitative analysis of the data obtained using DWI, ADC maps were generated from which ADC values of the ROIs were calculated according to the following equation:

$$ADC = \ln (S_0/S_1) (B_1 - B_0)$$

where S_0 and S_1 are signal intensities before and after application of diffusion gradients; B_1 and B_0 are the applied values. S_0 is the signal obtained in the spin echo sequence without using the gradient (b = 0 s/mm^2) and S_0 is obtained using the diffusion-attenuated MRI signal (b = 1000 s/mm^2).

MRI images were reviewed in consensus by two radiologists with 9 and 14 years' experience in breast MRI; both were blinded to clinical and histological findings except the presence of invasive breast cancer. In order to standardize and homologate image analysis as much as possible, the radiologists first reviewed subtracted images to identify the largest breast lesion. Additional lesions were considered only if measuring >5 mm. Multifocal carcinoma was diagnosed in the presence of multiple foci of malignancy in the same breast quadrant; multicentric carcinoma was diagnosed when two or more foci of malignancy were found in at least two quadrants; bilateral carcinoma was diagnosed if malignant lesions were found in both breasts (synchronous bilateral breast cancer)[12,13].

In case of multifocal disease, the primary index lesion was selected as the largest enhanced neoplastic mass identified on the subtracted images. Tumors were divided into two groups according to the size ($\leq$2 cm and >2 cm).

Subtracted images were subsequently superimposed on DWI images (b = 1000 s/mm^2) and on the ADC maps to detect cancer lesions. ADC value was obtained from the largest lesion by manually drawing a circular ROI measuring 3-6 mm in diameter on the slice where the lesion was most clearly visible. The circle was drawn around the enhanced solid portion to avoid areas of T2 shine-through, i.e. the necrotic core of the tumor, which appears hyperintense on ADC maps and hypointense on subtracted images. ADC value was automatically calculated.

47

4. Histological analysis

Specimens obtained by core biopsy or after surgery were submitted to histological analysis carried out by a pathologist with more than 15 years' experience. Analysis was performed in accordance with the WHO guidelines for tumor histotype classification: ductal, lobular, tubular carcinoma, etc.

In addition to grading, immunohistochemical test (IHC) was performed to evaluate molecular receptors (ER, PgR and HER2) and for Ki-67index calculation.

Hormone status for both steroid hormones, i.e. estrogen and progesterone, was assessed using Dako monoclonal antibody, dilution 1:100. Only nuclear reactivity was taken into account for ER. HER2 status was assessed according to recently published guidelines [14][14] using the Hercep Test (Dako, Glostrup, Denmark).

Samples yielding an equivocal IHC result were submitted to fluorescence in situ hybridization (FISH) analysis: a HER2 gene signal response localized on chromosome 17 exceeding 2.2 was used as a cut-off value to define HER2-gene amplification. Mib-1 monoclonal antibody (1:200 dilution; Dako, Glostrup, Denmark) was used to assess Ki-67 expression, which was reported as the percentage of immunoreactive cells out of 2,000 tumor cells randomly selected from the core of the tumor.

Hormone receptor status was considered to be positive if the expression was $\geq 10\%$ and negative if the expression was $<10\%$. HER2 expression was classified as follows: 0, 1+, 2+ or 3+; tumors reaching a score of 2+ or 3+ were considered to be HER2-positive whereas 0 or 1+ was considered to be HER2-negative. Ki-67 cut-off percentage was 14%; tumors with Ki-67 $\geq 14\%$ were considered to have a high rate of proliferative activity and those with $<14\%$ were considered to have a low rate proliferative activity.

5. Statistical analysis

For the statistical analysis, ADC was considered as a continuous dependent variable, whereas tumor grade was considered as an independent discrete variable. Kolmogorov-Smirnov test was performed to determine if ADC values followed a normal (or Gaussian) distribution and therefore to guide the choice of statistical subsequence test. The outcome of this test shows the statistical significance of the sampling distribution: if the significance level is greater than 0.05, sampling distribution is considered to be normal, whereas a significance level less than 0.05 indicates non-normal sampling distribution. If the ADC value does not follow a normal distribution[15], the analysis cannot be carried out using common parametric tests, such as the Student's t and ANOVA tests for analysis of variance. In that case analysis is carried out using non-parametric tests, such as Wilcoxon-Mann-Whitney and Kruskal-Wallis which require subdivision of the continuous variable in intervals or ranges. ADC was a parameter for non-Gaussian distribution (Sig <0.05), and statistical comparison between ADC values and grading was therefore carried out using both the above mentioned non-parametric tests: Wilcoxon-Mann-Whitney U test (two-group comparisons) and the Kruskal-Wallis H test (two or multiple-group comparisons). To emphasize the importance and the central role of grading as a prognostic factor, Spearman's Rho correlation test was carried out to evaluate if there was correlation between grading and other prognostic factors, such as tumor size, and organic factors, such as hormone receptor status, HER2 expression and Ki-67 proliferation index.

Pearson's chi-square test was carried out to compare the prognostic factors (tumor size, hormone receptor status, HER2 expression and Ki-67 index) obtained in the two extreme groups (G1 e G3) in order to establish if these features were significantly different.

Statistical significance was set at $p < 0.05$. Analysis of data was carried out using SPSS© statistical software program version 18.0.

Results

From April 2011 to January 2014, 451 pre-surgical breast DCE-MRI
examinations were performed for local staging. Patients were selected for the study
according to specific criteria as described under Materials and Methods, and a total of
359 were excluded: 186 because MRI was performed on 1.5 T, 99 because no
pathological confirmation was available; 42 because the patients had benign lesions
or ductal carcinoma in situ (CIS), five because the lesions were not visible on DWI
sequences, three because DWI sequences showed motion or distortion artifacts and
24 because ADC value was not assessed. A total of 96 breast lesions in 92 patients (4
patients had bilateral breast cancer) with histologically proven invasive breast cancer
were included in the study and their MRI scans were reviewed. Mean age of the
patients was 57.4 years (range 29-88 years); 45 patients (51.2%) were in menopause,
43 (48.8%) were premenopausal.

Revision of breast MRI scans revealed the characteristics summarized in Table 7.

Lesions (n =)	96
Margins	
Regular	2
Irregular	37
Lobulated	10
Spiculated	47
Enhancement	
Homogeneous	3
Heterogeneous	80
Peripheral with a central core	23
Kinetic curves	
Progressive (type I)	6
Plateau (type II)	47
Rapid wash-out (type III)	43

Size (median; mm)	17.16 (6-120)
Distribution of lesions	
Unifocal	53
Multifocal	20
Multicentric	12
Bilateral	11
T2 signal intensity	
Hyperintense	10
Hypointense/isointense	86

Table 7: Features revealed at breast MRI

Histopathological analysis showed that 73 lesions were invasive ductal carcinomas and 23 were lobular invasive carcinomas. As regards histological grading, 32 lesions were G1, 24 were G2 and 40 were G3. Immunohistochemical test revealed 77 ER-positive (80.2%) and 19 ER-negative tumors (19.8%); 73 PgR-positive (76%) and 23 PgR-negative tumors (24%); 23 HER2-positive (24%) and 73 HER2-negative tumors (76%). Ki-67 labeling index was ≥14% in 63 tumors (65.6%) and <14% in 33 tumors (34.4%).

Histopathological and immunohistochemical results are shown in Table 8.

Histological features	Lesions (n=)
Grading	
G1	32
G2	24
G3	40
ER +	77
ER -	19
PgR +	73
PgR -	23
HER2 +	23

HER2 -	73
Ki-67 +	63
Ki-67 -	33
Histotype	
Ductal	73
Lobular	23

Table 8: *Histopathological and immunohistochemical features of the lesions.*

The Kolmogorov-Smirnov test showed that the ADC values did not follow a normal distribution (p<0.05) (Fig. 7 and Table 9).

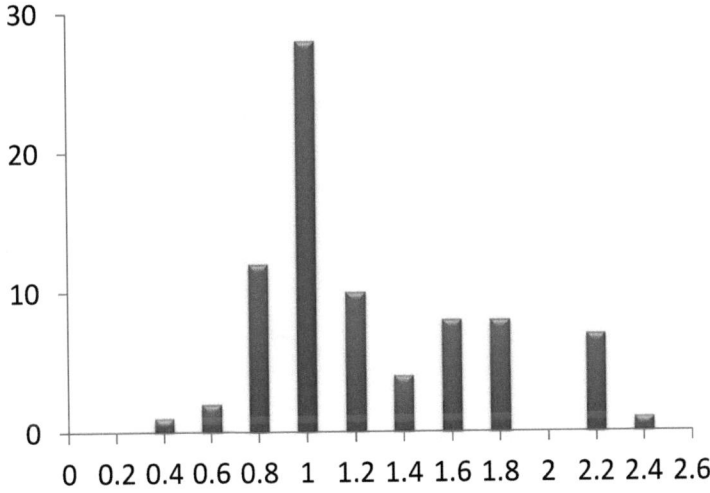

Figura 7: *The Kolmogorov-Smirnov test.*

	Values	df	Sig.
ADC	0.174	96	0. 014*10^{-5}

Table 9: *Statistical significance of the Kolmogorov-Smirnov test*

df: data frequency

Sig: significance

The Wilcoxon-Mann-Whitney test and the Kruskal-Wallis test showed that the ADC values were significantly higher in G1 tumors (ADC median value was 1.16, range 0.89-2.24) than in G3 tumors (ADC mean value was 1.03, range 0.45-1.77); statistical significance in both parametric tests was 0.037 (Fig. 8).

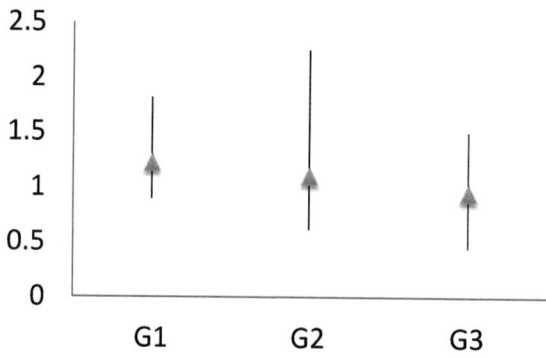

Fig. 8: *ADC values in the three groups*

No significant differences were found when the following groups were compared using a multivariable analysis: G2 vs G3 (p= 0.47), G1 vs G2 (p=0.126), and G1 vs G2 vs G3 (p=0.123).

Spearman's Rho correlation test demonstrated that tumor size correlated significantly with grading (Rho=0.456; p<0.001). A significant correlation was found also between molecular receptor expression and grading: for ER and PgR, Rho was 0.419 and 0.426, respectively, (p<0.001) and for HER2, Rho was 0.270 (p=0.08).

Also Ki-67 index correlated significantly with grading (Rho=0.489; p<0.001) (Fig. 9).

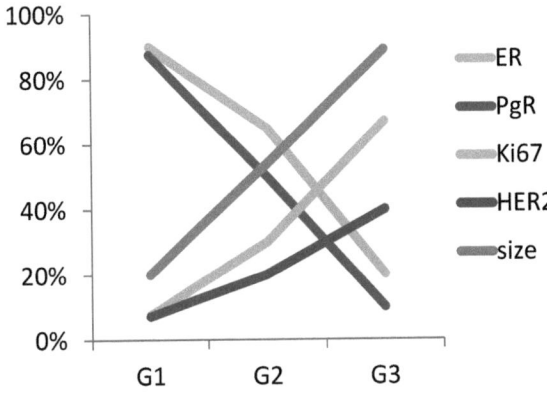

Fig. 9: Spearman's Rho correlation test

Correlation between the two extreme grades (G1 and G3) and the other prognostic factors yielded the following results: in G1, 27 lesions measured <2cm (84.4%) and five measured ≥2cm (15.6%); 32 lesions were ER-positive (100%) and 30 were PgR-positive (93.7%); there were no HER2-positive tumors (0%) and Ki-67 index was >14% in 6 lesions (18.7%). In G3, 13 lesions measured <2 cm (32.5%) and 27 measured ≥ 2 cm (67.5%); 24 lesions were ER-positive (60%) and 22 lesions were PgR-positive (55%); 14 tumors were HER2-positive (35%) and Ki-67 index was ≥ 14% in 35 lesions (87.5%).

Pearson's chi square test demonstrated that there was a significant difference between G1 and G3 related to the prognostic factors: ER and PgR status (p<0.01 and p=0.031, respectively), HER2 expression (p<0.01) and Ki-67 index (p=0.012). No statistically significant difference was observed in lesion size between the two groups (p=0.224) (Fig. 10).

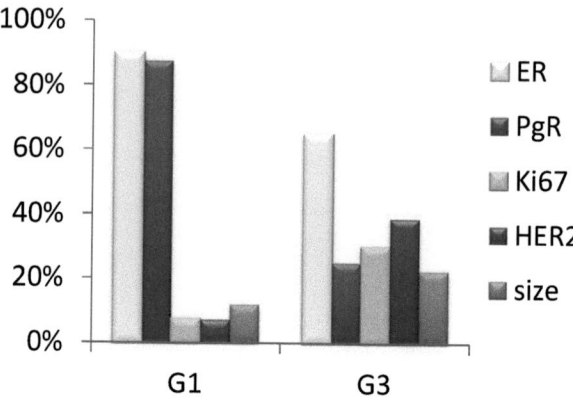

Fig. 10: *Pearson's chi square test: comparison of mean values.*

Discussion

DWI is a new accurate MRI technique which yields information about possible changes in the biological environment caused by development of lesions, whether malignant or benign. This method has shown elevated sensitivity in several diagnostic fields, as it can identify changes within the tissues by registering the Brownian motion of free water molecules. Water molecule motion is influenced by the local cellularity and the presence of possible obstacles, such as defective cell membranes and semipermeable membranes. Water molecule diffusion is impeded or blocked in tissues with a high cellular density (e.g. tumor tissue) but the motion is faster in an environment containing fewer cells and defective cell membranes (e.g. the necrotic portion of a large lesion). The degree of water diffusion in soft tissue is thus inversely correlated with tissue cellularity and the quality of healthy cell membranes.

However, water molecule diffusion is also greatly affected by other factors, such as viscosity of the intracellular and extracellular tissue fluids, active transport across the cell membranes, flow structure and direction of the flow[11]. Several studies have demonstrated that malignant lesions with altered features as described above, present higher signal intensity on DWI than benign breast lesions and normal fibroglandular tissue. Signal intensity on DWI is thus proportional to the degree of free water molecule mobility [16-21]. Intensity is quantified by measuring the ADC value, which expresses the average motion of a molecule per time unit measured in s/mm2; same ADC value is inversely proportional to signal intensity on DWI. As previously pointed out, the degree of enhancement is influenced by the histological structure of the tissues. Lesions with dense cellularity thus yield a hyperintense signal and lower ADC values. In contrast, low-density lesions are hypointense on DWI and present higher ADC values.

To date, diagnosis of malignancy has been made on the basis of histological outcome, which affects prognosis and guides therapeutic approach. Depending on the prognostic factors, such as histotype, histological grade, hormone and HER2 receptor status, degree of proliferation and tumor size, the clinicians decide if the patient should be submitted to surgery, chemotherapy, hormone therapy or a combination of these treatments.

Certain biological prognostic factors, such as hormone receptors and HER2 expression are now well established in terms of prognostic relevance and long-term results. However, a growing number of studies recognize the limitations of these factors in the overall prediction of malignant tumor evolution. It has been suggested that biological factors alone do not form a sufficiently reliable basis for management decisions in all patients. This concept has led to the need for additional parameters, such as grading.

NGS is currently the most commonly used system for malignant tumor grading. It is recommended by several international organizations, such as WHO, AJCC, EU and UK RCPath[42,43]. NGS establishes histological grading on the basis of three features: the presence of tubular structures, nuclear pleomorphism and mitotic count. Each feature is given a score ranging from 1 to 3, respectively; the scores are then added up to give a final total score ranging from 3-9. The role of NGS as an independent prognostic factor in breast cancer has been confirmed by several authors[12,43,44] and some have reported its prognostic value as equivalent to that of nodal status[45] and found it even more accurate than tumor size[43,46, 47]. NGS is furthermore a simple, inexpensive and easy way to assess the biological features of the tumor. Histological grading can accurately predict the evolution and response to therapy as well as prognosis. Some studies have in fact demonstrated that grading is a very important, independent prognostic factor in some specific breast cancer subgroups, e.g. in patients with ER-positive tumors[48] and particularly ER-positive tumors in the absence of HER2 receptor expression.

Grading seems to have a fundamental role in defining the prognosis of small tumors. Rakha et al.[46] reported that recurrence was very rare in patients with G1 tumors. Relapse occurred in patients with a higher-grade tumor; otherwise the lesion was found to be a second primary tumor Development of metastases and death were rare events (4%) in patients with tumors classified G1 unless they developed a second primary tumor of a higher grade[49]. This observation implies that most G1 tumors carry a low risk of adverse events. Therefore, if the grading is not taken into consideration, these tumors may be overtreated asthe risk of adverse events might be overestimated.

In this context, Rakha et al. underlined the important association between histological grade and long-term survival. High-grade tumors tend to recur and metastasize early, typically within the first eight years of the onset until death. Low-grade tumors have a good outcome; adverse events, such as recurrence and metastases, are few and have little or no effect. This means that low-grade tumors have a good prognosis, while high-grade tumors require immediate treatment, including chemotherapy, owing to the risk of early recurrence and death. Grading is essential also for the treatment planning, because fast-growing tumors (G3) are more likely to respond to chemotherapy than slow-growing tumors (G1).

Grade 2 tumors show an intermediate outcome during the early years of follow-up, but over time they tend to recur and metastasize in conjunction with evolution towards a less differentiated histological pattern. The last St. Gallen International Expert Consensus on the Primary Therapy of Early Breast Cancer (2009)[50] thus recommended that only G1 and G3 tumors should be considered for adjuvant chemotherapy. In this study, G2 tumors were not taken into consideration, as the intermediate values would have caused a lack of equilibrium in the statistical analysis and the comparison with the ADC values. Misassignment to G1 and G3 rarely occurs, whereas Grade 2 values are often subject to discordance between pathologists in the definition of the score. This is to be expected, since classification of samples is often difficult in lesions presenting overlapping areas. Grade 2 should actually be considered of intermediate value in risk assessment in line with other borderline outcomes, such as tumor size between 2 and 5 cm, poor lymph node involvement (1 out of 3) or borderline outcome of the genetic tests, which do not provide a clear indication as to the usefulness of neoadjuvant chemotherapy.

Scientific research is studying a new approach to "intermediate" tumors thanks to the possibilities offered by molecular profiling tests to be carried out in cases of diagnostic doubt[43]. The aim is to divide G2 tumors into two subgroups: one subgroup close to G1 which includes tumors with a good outcome that may not require adjuvant chemotherapy; the other subgroup close to G3 which includes tumors with a high risk of recurrence and metastases requiring chemotherapy after surgery.

Only a few studies using 1.5T MRI have evaluated the correlation between tumor grading and ADC values obtained from ADC maps provided by DWI[14,51]. In this study, comparison between ADC values and grading showed that histological grade influences the ADC values, and a significant difference was found between ADC values of the two extreme groups, G1 and G3.

This finding indicates the existence of a correlation between ADC values, DWI signal and some histological features, particularly those evaluated in the grading (tubular formation, mitotic count, the presence of tubular formations and the degree of atypia).This means that abundant proliferation, high mitotic activity and reduced tubular formation are signs of increased cellularity of the parenchyma as demonstrated by the elevated DWI signal intensity and low ADC value. The results obtained in this study are consistent with those reported in our recent retrospective analysis[52] as well as the studies published by Martincich et al. and Razek et al.[38,53]. They all confirm that ADC values may be a useful diagnostic tool for identifying biologically aggressive lesions.

No statistically significant difference was found between the grades correlated to the ADC values when also G2 was included in the statistical analysis. As previously pointed out, this was due to the fact that G2 tumors present intermediate morphological and biological features and thus also intermediate prognosis which causes distortion as the tumor features and aggressiveness are close to either G1 with

59

a good prognosis or G3 with a poor prognosis. This occurs because the histological technique used to evaluate the grading score involves semi-quantitative evaluation of the morphological features. G2 tumors, which have a score of 6-7, may often be close to G1 or G3. G2 tumors are therefore often subject to discordance between pathologists. In the statistical evaluation, G2 tumors did not show correlation with ADC values, and the subsequent statistical analysis was therefore carried out only on the two extreme groups (G1 and G3).

In order to test the significance acquired by this prognostic factor in the recent years, confirmed also by several scientific reports, and to assess the ability of grading to express the intrinsic biological features of the tumors, grading was correlated with other prognostic factors in breast cancer, such as tumor size and the biological factors ER, PgR and HER2 receptor status as well as Ki-67 index. Furthermore, in order to establish if the two extreme groups G1 and G3 presented significant differences, their individual relationships with the above mentioned prognostic factors were analyzed one by one and the outcomes were compared.

It is of interest to note that there was a significant difference between G1 and G3 related to ER and PR status, HER2 expression and Ki-67 index. G1 lesions were more often ER- and PgR-positive and HER2-negative with Ki-67 index <14%, whereas G3 lesions were more often ER and PgR-negative and HER2-positive with Ki-67 index >14%.

On the basis of these results, confirmed by Rakha et al., we affirm that grading is a comprehensive index of the intrinsic biological features of a tumor as it can accurately predict clinical behavior and consequent prognosis. Grading has been accused of a poor reproducibility and therefore of being inadequate as a prognostic factor. However, it now seems that the main reason for this limitation was incorrect harvesting and preservation of the samples. Suboptimal fixation causes a loss of cells and reduces the possibility to count mitotic figures and evaluate the nuclei. In this connection, the new guidelines for the standardization of pre-analytical parameters include recommendations for harvesting, fixation and sample preparation as well as assignment of score and grading. In this way, histological grade can become an important tool for choosing the most appropriate clinical management and for guiding the decision-making process as well as the choice of treatment.

In the literature, only a few studies deal with 3T MRI studies in which ADC values were compared to grading. The present study includes only patients who had undergone breast 3T MRI. The magnetic field strength of 3T MRI is medium-high. SNR and spatial resolution are therefore higher than those of low-field methods reported in the literature, such as 1.5T, but 3T MRI acquisition time is longer. Matsuoka et al.[54] reported a more accurate lesion delineation on DWI using 3T MRI compared to 1.5T, and they obtained a better visibility of tumors measuring <10 mm on 3T MRI compared to 1.5T.

On the other hand, the use of a high magnetic field strength leads to an increased number of artifacts, such as chemical shift and susceptibility artifacts in general, while impaired homogeneity of B_1 and B_0 may cause image distortion and inhomogeneous fat suppression[26].

In this study, greater susceptibility to artifacts and nonuniformity of the magnetic field were minimized by increasing the number of image acquisitions and increasing slice thickness. In order to reduce chemical shift artifacts, the largest dimension of the matrix was increased. Fat suppression was essential to reduce artifacts (e.g. ghosting and chemical shift artifacts) and to increase image conspicuity. Fat suppression was obtained by inversion recovery sequences using a 180 degree RF pulse and a short inversion time (short time inversion recovery - STIR sequences) before acquisition of echo-planar DWI sequences. STIR sequences have the disadvantage of a lower SNR, but they provide a more uniform fat suppression, which is essential to reduce artifacts and increase image conspicuity. All MRI scans performed in this study were of a satisfactory diagnostic quality, except in 3 cases due to motion artifacts. Moreover, as previously mentioned, some authors have observed that small lesions are more clearly visible on 3T MRI[54].

In order to standardize the setting of the magnetic field for image acquisition as much as possible, only b 1000 sec/mm^2 was used in all patients. Pereira et al. reported that it was not necessary to use multiple b-values, because the sensitivity of the ADC value obtained by using two b-values was equivalent to the value obtained using multiple b-values. Therefore, also in view of the time constraints existing in clinical practice, the analysis of ADC using two b-values should be considered acceptable.

In order to minimize the effects of inter-observer variation, ROI was positioned on the ADC map in the region corresponding to the lesion that appeared most vascularized on the subtracted images (Fig. 2) superimposing the two images while avoiding the necrotic portion.

This study has some limitations:

- It was retrospectively performed in a single institution;

- The sample size was relatively small; larger scale studies are required to produce more reliable ADC values for evaluating breast malignancies;

- Correlation between grading and ADC may have been influenced by some histological features of the tumors, such as angiogenesis and necrosis, which influence the motility of water molecules and thereby DWI signal intensity[55,56];

- ROI selection may have influenced our results; ROI was determined by superimposing subtracted images on DWI images in the most vascularized portion of the lesion avoiding the necrotic areas. ADC values may thus have been significantly influenced by microperfusion and they may therefore not reliably reflect the cellularity of the lesion. In order to obtain clinically useful ADC values, the best measuring method should be identified for each type of lesion, especially in the presence of mixed tumor patterns.

Despite these limitations, we believe that accurate ADC values were obtained in this study thanks to improved SNR and contrast-to-noise ratios provided by the 3T MRI scanner.

Conclusions

Our findings suggest that ADC values found in invasive breast cancer lesions obtained on 3T DWI images, correlate significantly with G1 and G3 histological tumor grades. A significant difference was found between G1 and G3 relative to the expression of some biological and histological factors, such as ER, PgR and HER2 receptor status and Ki-67 index. In comparison with G1 lesions, G3 lesions were more often ER- and PgR-negative, HER2-positive and with a Ki-67 index >14%.

Some authors have suggested that the TNM staging system, which evaluates the anatomical extent of the tumor, should be associated with grading, which can improve assessment by adding histological features reflecting the probability of metastatic dissemination and death. In this diagnostic procedure, MRI is a highly accurate imaging technique which can provide morphological evaluation and show tumor extent. Moreover, MRI provides ADC values obtained on DWI sequences thereby constituting a useful tool for the integration of biological features of invasive breast cancer required to guide management and predict clinical behavior and prognosis

Further studies of 3T MRI imaging in larger patient populations are required to assess the value of ADC value as an independent prognostic factor.

References

1. Kumar V, Abbas A.K, Fausto N AJC. Robins e Cotran. Le basi patologiche delle malattie. Malattie degli organi e degli apparati. Vol. 2. *Elsevier*. 2008. Available at: http://www.libreriauniversitaria.it/robbins-cotran-basi-patologiche-malattie/libro/9788821431753. Accessed July 6, 2014.

2. Bassett LW, Dhaliwal SG, Eradat J, et al. National trends and practices in breast MRI. *AJR Am J Roentgenol*. 2008;191(2):332-9. doi:10.2214/AJR.07.3207.

3. Sardanelli F, Boetes C, Borisch B, et al. Magnetic resonance imaging of the breast: recommendations from the EUSOMA working group. *Eur J Cancer*. 2010;46(8):1296-316. doi:10.1016/j.ejca.2010.02.015.

4. Mann RM, Hoogeveen YL, Blickman JG, Boetes C. MRI compared to conventional diagnostic work-up in the detection and evaluation of invasive lobular carcinoma of the breast: a review of existing literature. *Breast cancer Res Treat*. 2008;107(1):1-14.

5. Gordon Y, Partovi S, Müller-Eschner M, et al. Dynamic contrast-enhanced magnetic resonance imaging: fundamentals and application to the evaluation of the peripheral perfusion. *Cardiovasc Diagn Ther*. 2014;4(2):147-164. doi:10.3978/j.issn.2223-3652.2014.03.01.

6. Amarnath J, Sangeeta T, Mehta SB. Role of quantitative pharmacokinetic parameter (transfer constant: K(trans)) in the characterization of breast lesions on MRI. *Indian J Radiol Imaging*. 2013;23(1):19-25. doi:10.4103/0971-3026.113614.

7. Vanzulli A, Torricelli P, Colagrande S, Cova M.A GM. Manuale di RM per TSRM (Tecnici di Radiologia Medica) [Vanzulli; Torricelli - Poletto] - Risonanza Magnetica - Diagnostica per Immagini - Medicina. *Polet Ed*. 2013. Available at: http://www.medicalinformation.it/ecommerce/manuale-di-rm-per-tsrm-vanzulli-torricelli-poletto-9788895033525vanzulli-angelo-torricelli-pietro-colagrande-stefano-cova-maria-assunta-gallucci-massimo.html. Accessed July 6, 2014.

8. Kuhl CK, Gieseke J, von Falkenhausen M, et al. Sensitivity encoding for diffusion-weighted MR imaging at 3.0 T: intraindividual comparative study. *Radiology*. 2005;234(2):517-26. doi:10.1148/radiol.2342031626.

9. Elston C, Ellis I. Pathological prognostic factors in breast cancer. I. The value of histological grade in breast cancer: experience from a large study with long-term follow-up. *Histopathology*. 1991;(19):403-410.

10. Hansemann D. Ueber asymmetrische Zelltheilung in Epithelkrebsen und deren biologische Bedeutung. *Arch für Pathol Anat und Physiol und für Klin Med.* 1890;119(2):299-326. doi:10.1007/BF01882039.

11. Greenough RB. Varying Degrees of Malignancy in Cancer of the Breast. *J Cancer Res.* 1925;9(4):453-463. doi:10.1158/jcr.1925.453.

12. Macis D, Cazzaniga M, De Censi a, Bonanni B. Role of traditional and new biomarkers in breast carcinogenesis. *Ecancermedicalscience.* 2009;3:157. doi:10.3332/ecancer.2009.157.

13. Van Diest PJ, van der Wall E, Baak JP a. Prognostic value of proliferation in invasive breast cancer: a review. *J Clin Pathol.* 2004;57(7):675-81. doi:10.1136/jcp.2003.010777.

14. Martincich L, Deantoni V, Bertotto I, et al. Correlations between diffusion-weighted imaging and breast cancer biomarkers. *Eur Radiol.* 2012;22(7):1519-28. doi:10.1007/s00330-012-2403-8.

15. Razali NM, Wah YB. Power comparisons of Shapiro-Wilk , Kolmogorov-Smirnov , Lilliefors and Anderson-Darling tests. *J Stat Model Anal.* 2011;2(1):21-33.

16. Kim SH, Cha ES, Kim HS, et al. Diffusion-weighted imaging of breast cancer: correlation of the apparent diffusion coefficient value with prognostic factors. *J Magn Reson Imaging.* 2009;30(3):615-20. doi:10.1002/jmri.21884.

17. Guo Y, Cai Y-Q, Cai Z-L, et al. Differentiation of clinically benign and malignant breast lesions using diffusion-weighted imaging. *J Magn Reson Imaging.* 2002;16(2):172-8. doi:10.1002/jmri.10140.

18. Park MJ, Cha ES, Kang BJ, Ihn YK, Baik JH. The role of diffusion-weighted imaging and the apparent diffusion coefficient (ADC) values for breast tumors. *Korean J Radiol.* 2007;8(5):390-6. Available at: http://www.pubmedcentral.nih.gov/articlerender.fcgi?artid=2626812&tool=pmcentr ez&rendertype=abstract. Accessed April 27, 2014.

19. Partridge SC, Mullins CD, Kurland BF, et al. Apparent diffusion coefficient values for discriminating benign and malignant breast MRI lesions: effects of lesion type and size. *AJR Am J Roentgenol.* 2010;194(6):1664-73. doi:10.2214/AJR.09.3534.

20. Marini C, Iacconi C, Giannelli M, Cilotti A, Moretti M, Bartolozzi C. Quantitative diffusion-weighted MR imaging in the differential diagnosis of breast lesion. *Eur Radiol.* 2007;17(10):2646-55. doi:10.1007/s00330-007-0621-2.

21. Jeh SK, Kim SH, Kim HS, et al. Correlation of the apparent diffusion coefficient value and dynamic magnetic resonance imaging findings with prognostic factors in invasive ductal carcinoma. *J Magn Reson Imaging*. 2011;33(1):102-9. doi:10.1002/jmri.22400.

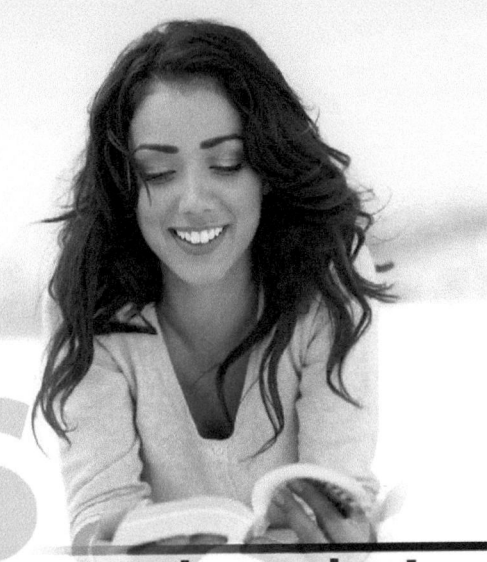
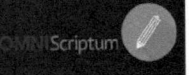

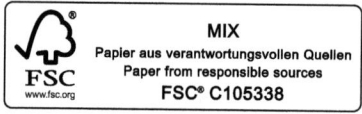
Printed by Books on Demand GmbH, Norderstedt / Germany